FLEXIBILITY AT ANY AGE

CHAIR YOGA FOR MEN OVER 50

By

Joseph T. Shea

TABLE OF CONTENTS

INTRODUCTION:

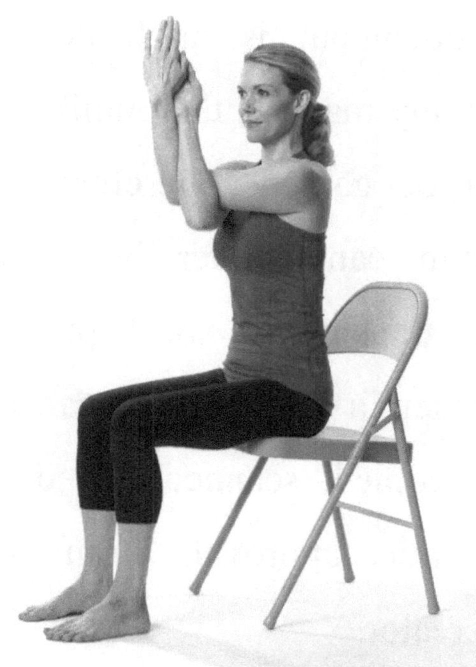

Welcome to the transformative world of chair yoga, where age is just a number and flexibility knows no bounds. In this

6

comprehensive guide, we embark on a journey of self-discovery and holistic well-being, exploring the power of chair yoga to unlock vitality, resilience, and joy in the lives of men over 50. Whether you're a seasoned yogi or a complete novice, this book is your gateway to a healthier, happier, and more flexible future.

UNDERSTANDING CHAIR YOGA

Let's begin by demystifying the concept of chair yoga. What exactly is chair yoga, and how does it differ from traditional yoga? At its core, chair yoga is a gentle form of yoga that adapts traditional poses and practices to be performed while seated or using a chair for support. It offers all the benefits of traditional yoga—improved flexibility, strength, balance, and mental clarity—while making the practice accessible to individuals with mobility limitations, injuries, or other health concerns.

BENEFITS OF CHAIR YOGA FOR MEN OVER 50

Why chair yoga specifically for men over 50? As we age, our bodies undergo various changes—muscles may weaken, joints may stiffen, and balance may become less steady. Chair yoga offers a safe and effective way for men in this demographic to address these physical changes, maintain or improve their flexibility, and support overall health and well-being. Beyond the physical benefits, chair yoga also provides opportunities for stress relief, relaxation, and mental clarity—qualities that are especially valuable in the fast-paced modern world.

PRINCIPLES AND PRACTICES OF CHAIR YOGA

At its heart, chair yoga is about more than just physical exercise—it's a holistic practice that integrates body, mind, and spirit. In this book, we'll explore the core principles and practices of chair yoga, including mindful movement, breath awareness, and relaxation techniques. We'll learn how to synchronize breath with movement, cultivate presence and awareness in each pose, and create a sense of calm and balance that extends beyond the mat and into everyday life.

SETTING UP FOR SUCCESS

Before we dive into the world of chair yoga, let's take a moment to set ourselves up for success. Creating a comfortable and inviting space for your practice is essential. Find a quiet, clutter-free area where you can move freely without distractions. Choose a sturdy chair with a flat seat and firm backrest—avoid chairs with wheels or armrests that restrict movement. Place your chair on a nonslip surface, such as a yoga mat or carpet, to prevent it from sliding during your practice.

GETTING STARTED WITH CHAIR YOGA POSES

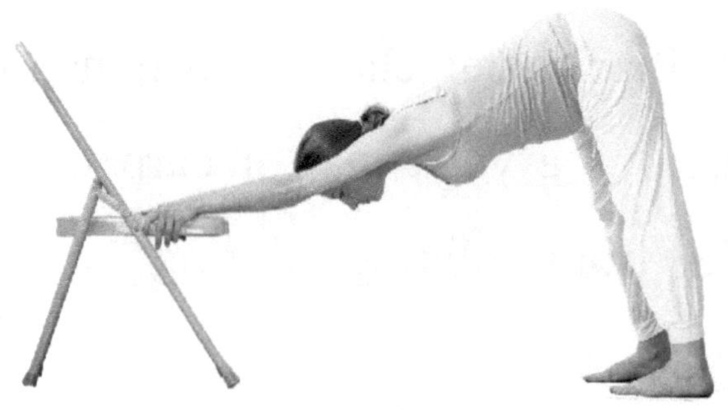

Now that we've set the stage, it's time to get started with some basic chair yoga poses. We'll begin with gentle warm-up exercises to awaken the body and prepare it for movement. From there, we'll progress to a series of seated poses that target different areas of the body—neck, shoulders, spine, hips, and legs—helping to improve flexibility, mobility, and range of motion. Throughout the practice, remember to listen to your body, honor its limits, and modify or skip any poses that feel uncomfortable or unsafe.

BREATH AWARENESS AND RELAXATION TECHNIQUES

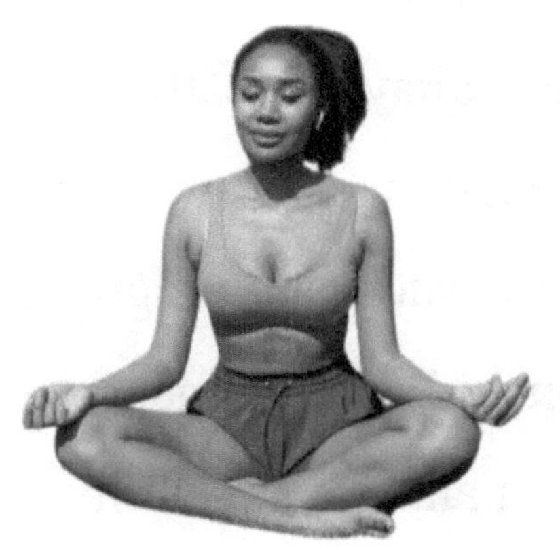

Breath is the bridge between body and mind, the anchor that keeps us grounded and present in the moment. In chair yoga, breath awareness is key—it helps to synchronize movement with breath, deepen the relaxation response, and cultivate a sense of inner peace and tranquility. We'll explore various breathing techniques, such as deep belly breathing, ujjayi breath, and alternate nostril breathing, as well as relaxation techniques, such as progressive muscle relaxation and guided imagery, to promote stress relief and mental clarity.

CULTIVATING MINDFULNESS IN PRACTICE

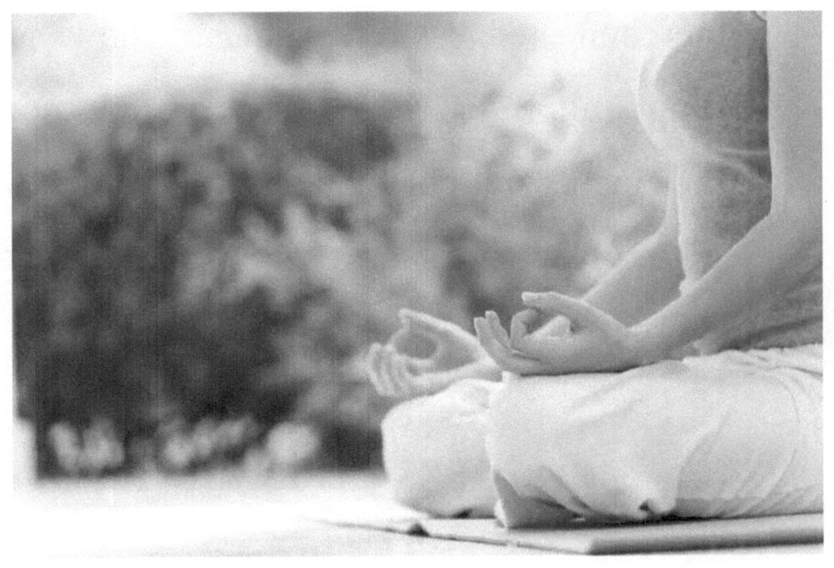

As we move through our chair yoga practice, we'll cultivate mindfulness—a state of open-hearted awareness and acceptance of the present moment. Mindfulness allows us to deepen our connection to ourselves, others, and the world around us, fostering a sense of peace, compassion, and interconnectedness. We'll learn how to bring mindfulness to our breath, our movement, and our thoughts, cultivating a sense of spaciousness and ease in body and mind.

PROGRESSING IN YOUR PRACTICE

As you continue on your chair yoga journey, you may find yourself wanting to explore more advanced poses and practices. In this book, we'll provide guidance on how to progress in your practice safely and effectively, building strength, flexibility, and confidence over time. We'll explore challenging variations and modifications for experienced practitioners, as well as opportunities to deepen your understanding of yoga philosophy and spirituality. Remember, yoga is a lifelong journey—there's always more to learn, explore, and discover.

CHAPTER 1:

UNDERSTANDING CHAIR YOGA

Welcome to Chapter 1 of "Flexibility at Any Age: Chair Yoga for Men Over 50." In this chapter, we'll delve into the fundamentals of chair yoga, exploring what it is, how it differs from traditional yoga, and why it's uniquely suited for men over 50. So, let's roll up our sleeves, or rather, settle comfortably into our chairs, and begin our journey of discovery.

WHAT IS CHAIR YOGA?

At its core, chair yoga is a gentle form of yoga that adapts traditional poses and practices to be performed while seated or using a chair for support. It offers all the benefits of traditional yoga—improved flexibility, strength, balance, and mental clarity—while making the practice accessible to individuals with mobility limitations, injuries, or other health concerns. Chair yoga is inclusive and welcoming, catering to practitioners of all ages, abilities, and fitness levels.

HOW IS CHAIR YOGA DIFFERENT?

You may be wondering: What sets chair yoga apart from traditional yoga? While both forms of yoga share many similarities—such as breath awareness, mindful movement, and relaxation techniques—chair yoga offers a unique approach to practice. By utilizing a chair for support, stability, and balance, chair yoga allows practitioners to perform a wide range of poses and movements safely and comfortably, without the need to get down on the floor or perform weight-bearing activities. This makes chair yoga particularly well-suited for individuals with limited mobility, joint pain, or other physical challenges.

BENEFITS FOR MEN OVER 50

Now, let's explore why chair yoga is especially beneficial for men over 50. As we age, our bodies undergo various changes—muscles may weaken, joints may stiffen, and balance may become less steady. Chair yoga offers a safe and effective way for men in this demographic to address these physical changes, maintain or improve their flexibility, and support overall health and well-being. Beyond the physical benefits, chair yoga also provides opportunities for stress relief, relaxation, and mental clarity—

qualities that are especially valuable in the fast-paced modern world.

ACCESSIBILITY AND INCLUSIVITY

One of the key strengths of chair yoga is its accessibility and inclusivity. Unlike traditional yoga, which often requires practitioners to perform poses on a mat or on the ground, chair yoga can be practiced almost anywhere, anytime—all you need is a sturdy chair and a little bit of space. This makes chair yoga ideal for individuals who may have difficulty getting up and down from the floor, such as older adults, individuals with disabilities, or those recovering from injury or surgery. Chair yoga invites everyone to participate in the transformative power of yoga, regardless of age, fitness level, or physical ability.

TAILORED TO INDIVIDUAL NEEDS
Another benefit of chair yoga is its adaptability and flexibility. Chair yoga poses and practices are readily adapted and tailored to individual requirements and tastes. Whether you're Yoga, and why it's especially beneficial for guys over 50. So, let us roll up our sleeves, or rather, sit down in our recliners, and begin our adventure of discovery.

GATEWAY TO MINDFULNESS

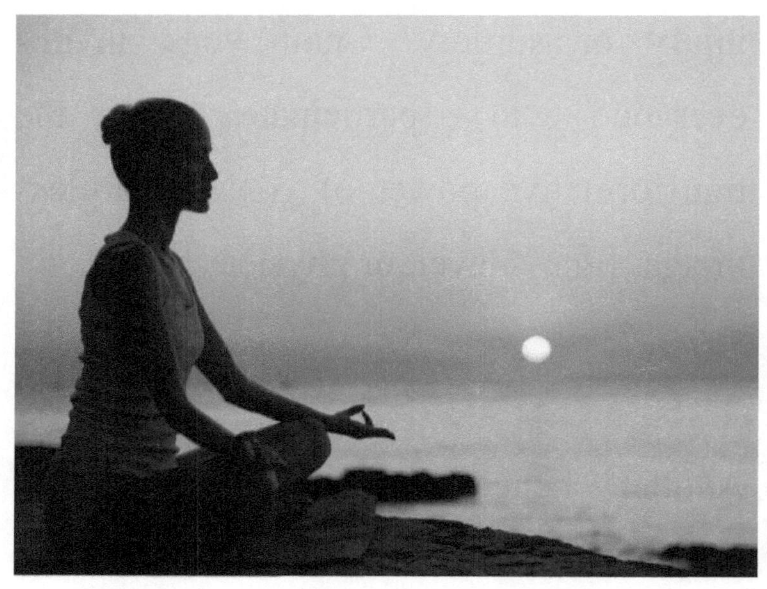

Aside from the physical benefits, chair yoga promotes mindfulness—a state of open-hearted awareness and acceptance of the present moment. Chair yoga fosters presence, attention, and inner quiet via breath awareness, mindful movement, and relaxation techniques. Chair yoga helps us to explore the rich tapestry of our inner experience by concentrating on physical sensations, breath rhythm, and mental fluctuations, resulting in a stronger connection with ourselves and the world around us.

 has provided us a solid foundation for understanding chair yoga. We've spoken about what chair yoga is, how it differs from conventional yoga, and why it's particularly beneficial to men over 50. We discovered its adaptability, accessibility, and transformative potential, as well as its invitation to mindfulness and self-awareness. Armed with this knowledge, we're ready to dive further into our chair yoga practice, finding the postures, concepts, and practices that will help us reach health, vitality, and flexibility in any age.

CHAPTER 2:

GETTING STARTED WITH CHAIR YOGA

In this chapter, we'll start our chair yoga journey by learning how to set up a comfortable practice location, learn basic chair yoga postures, and discover the transformative power of breathing and relaxation techniques. So let's roll up our sleeves, or rather, get comfortable in our seats, and begin exploring chair yoga.

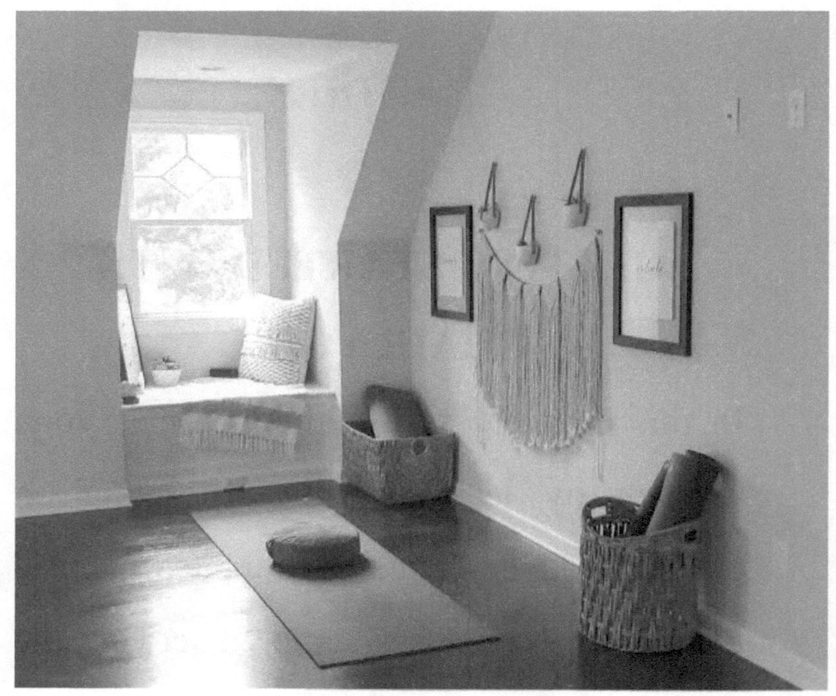

Before we begin our chair yoga practice, let's take a moment to prepare. Creating a nice and appealing environment for your practice is essential. Find a serene, clutter-free environment in which you may move freely and without interruption. Select a

28

sturdy chair with a flat seat and firm backrest; avoid chairs with wheels or armrests that restrict movement. Place your chair on a nonslip surface, such as a yoga mat or carpet, to prevent it from slipping throughout your practice.

CLOTHING & ACCESSORIES

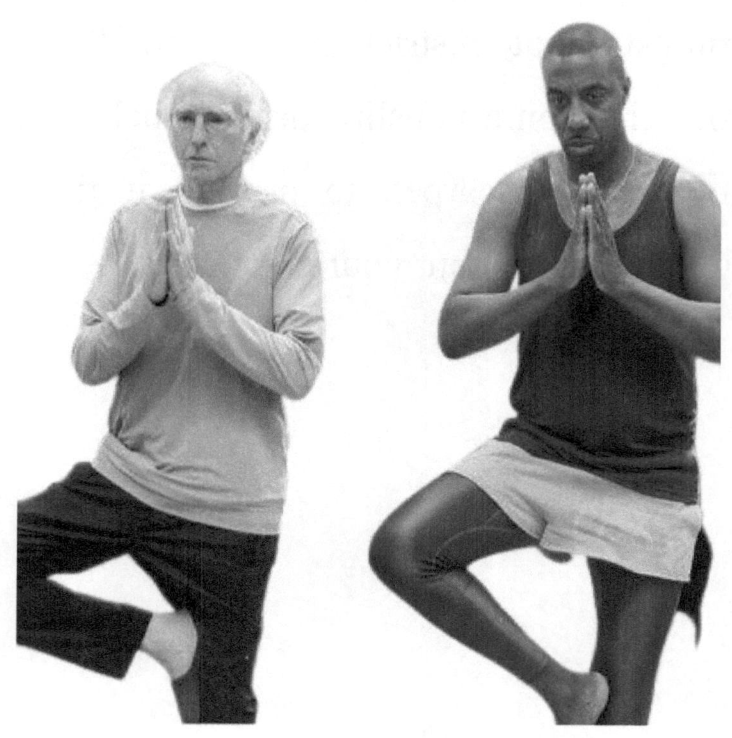

Dress casually and comfortably for chair yoga so that you may move freely and breathe deeply. Avoid wearing tight or confining apparel that may limit your motions or cause discomfort. Consider wearing layers that you may readily remove if you become too warm throughout your practice. You might also want to keep a small pillow or cushion nearby to assist support your back or knees as required.

WARM-UP EXERCISES.

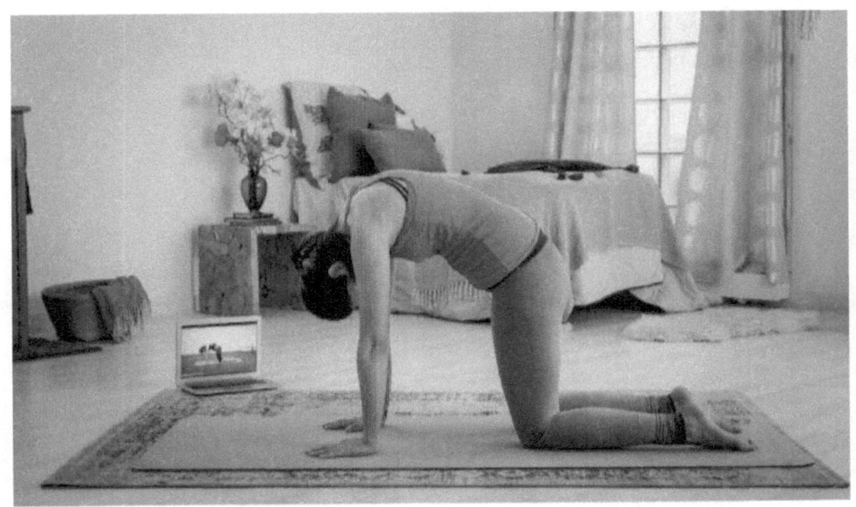

Let's begin our chair yoga practice with some gentle warm-up techniques to prepare the body for movement. Start by sitting comfortably on your chair, feet flat on the floor, spine tall and straight. Take a few deep breaths, inhaling with your nose and exhaling through your mouth, and let any tension or stress go away with each one.

NECK AND SHOULDER ROLLS.

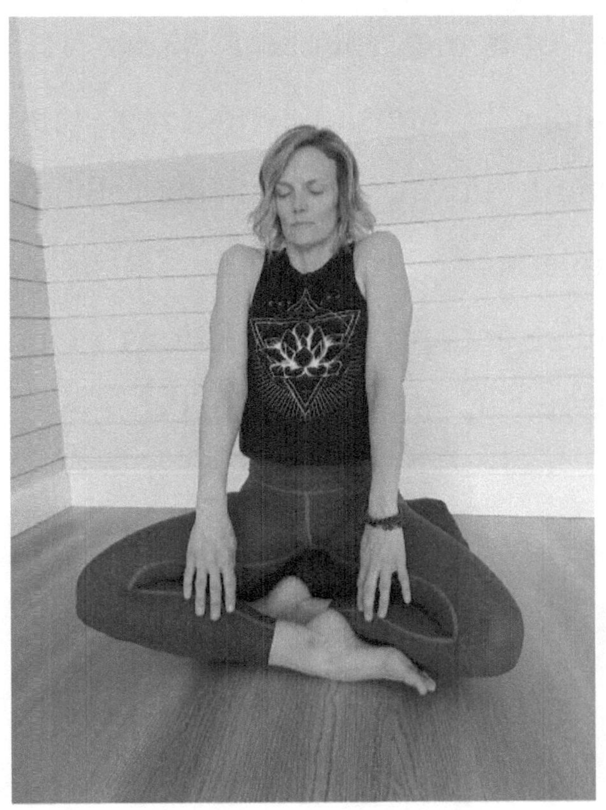

Begin by rotating your shoulders up, back, and down in a smooth, circular motion. Repeat this movement a few times, allowing your breath to determine the rhythm. Next, gently tilt your head to one side, bringing your ear closer to your shoulder, before slowly moving your head forward, down, and to the other side, completing a full circle. Repeat this exercise in opposite directions to relieve neck and shoulder strain and stiffness.

SEATED CAT-COW STRETCH

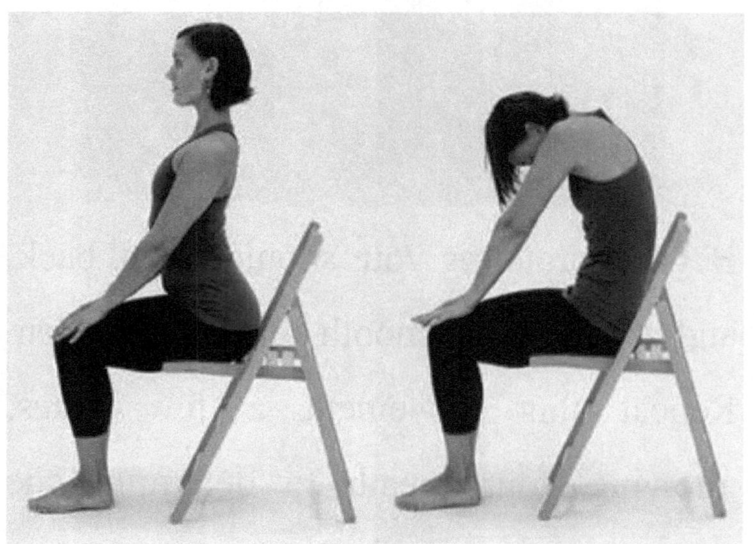

Next, we'll practice a seated variant of the well-known Cat-Cow Stretch to help move the spine and ease back tension. Begin by sitting upright in your chair, hands resting on your knees. As you inhale, arch your back and raise your chest to the ceiling, pulling your shoulder blades together and gazing upward. As you exhale, circle your back and tuck your chin into your chest, bringing your belly button towards your spine. Repeat the movement many times while breathing freely.

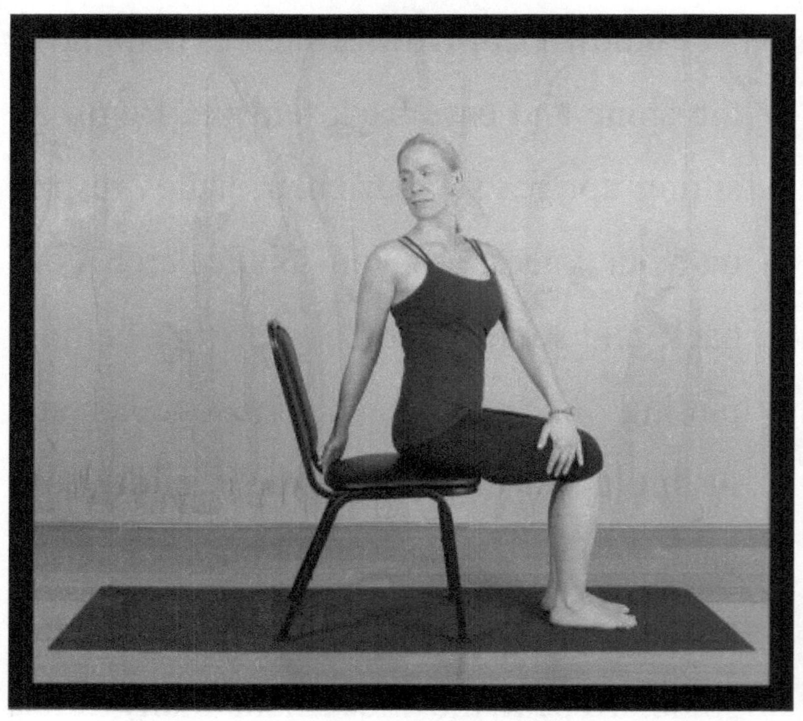

Now, perform a gentle Seated Side Stretch to stretch the sides of your body. Begin by sitting tall on your chair, feet flat on the floor and arms at your sides. As you inhale, raise your right arm to the heavens, extending through your fingertips, and then lean slightly to the left to create a long line of energy from your right fingertips to your left hip. Hold this stretch for a few breaths, feeling the sensation of stretching down your right side. Repeat on the opposite side, lifting your left arm to the ceiling and bending to the right.

SEATED FORWARD FOLD.

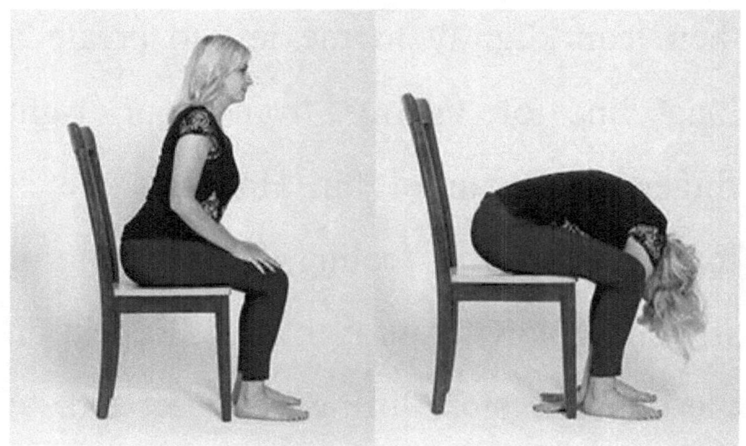

Finally, to reduce back and hamstring stress, execute a modest Seated Forward Fold exercise. Start by sitting tall on your chair, feet flat on the floor, and hands resting on your thighs. As you inhale, extend through the crown of your head; as you exhale, tilt forward from the hips, bringing your chest to your thighs and reaching your hands to your feet. Fold forward and long spine and relaxed neck, allowing gravity to increase the stretch in your back and hamstrings. Hold this posture for a few breaths before gently returning to the upright position.

BREATH AWARENESS

Remember to keep your breath in mind as you practice chair yoga. The breath is the cornerstone of yoga, controlling the movement and flow of energy throughout the body. Synchronize your breathing with your movement as you progress through each posture, inhaling deeply as you extend or lengthen and expelling completely as you contract or release.

Consider how the breath calms the mind, deepens the stretch, and cultivates a sense of presence and relaxation in the body.

RELAXATION TECHNIQUES

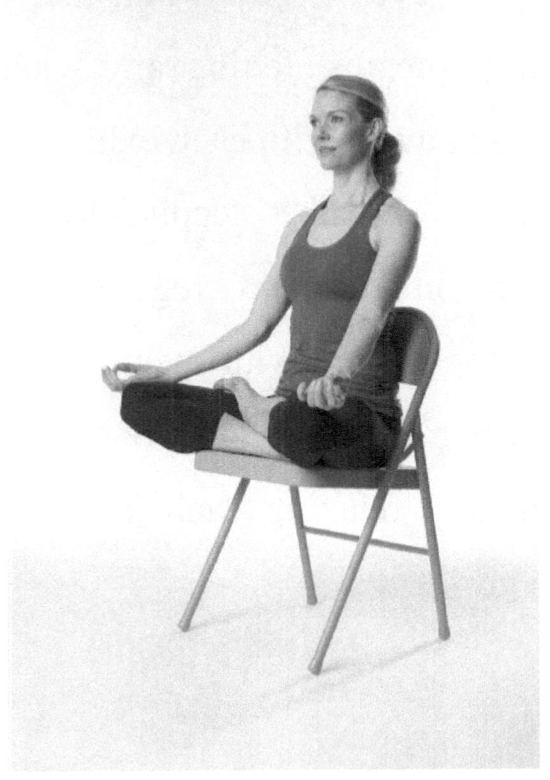

As we wrap up our chair yoga practice, let's take a time to decompress with some easy relaxation methods. Find a comfortable sitting posture in your chair, close your eyes if you want, and take a few deep breaths, letting any tension or worry melt away with each exhale. As you continue to breathe deeply, focus your attention on different regions of your body, beginning with your toes and progressing to the crown of your head, intentionally relaxing each muscle group as you go.

VISUALIZATION MEDITATION

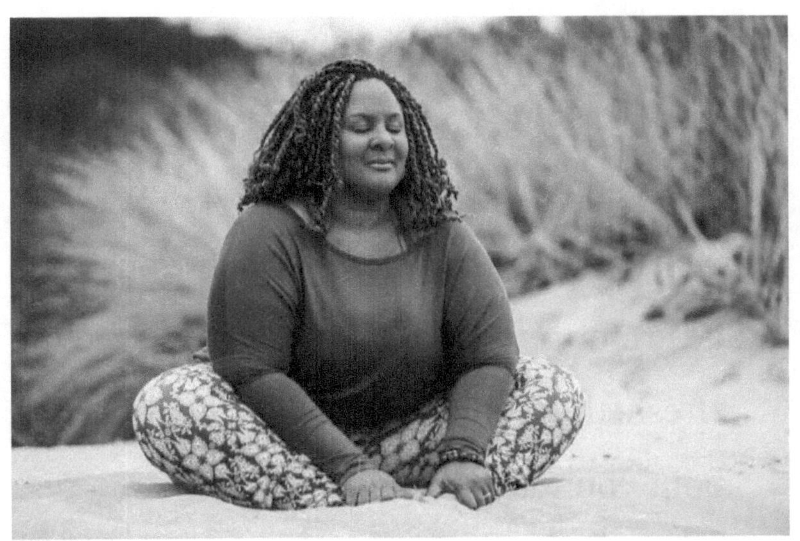

Finally, let's wrap off our practice with a little visualization meditation to encourage relaxation and inner calm. Imagine yourself sitting in a lovely, calm setting, such as a peaceful garden, a placid beach, or a quiet mountainside. As you breathe deeply, imagine the sights, sounds, and sensations of this area, allowing yourself to get completely involved in it. Feel a wave of serenity and tranquillity pour over you, encasing you in a warm embrace of peace and well-being. Take a few more deep breaths, then gently open your eyes and return to the present now, feeling refreshed, invigorated, and ready to go about your day.

CHAPTER 3

DEVELOPING STRENGTH AND FLEXIBILITY

Welcome to Chapter Three of "Flexibility at Any Age: Chair Yoga for Men Over 50." In this chapter, we'll look at how chair yoga may help you gain strength and flexibility, which are both important components of general health and well-being. We'll go through a sequence of gentle postures and mindful movements to improve mobility, range of motion, and build a feeling of balance and stability in both the body and mind. So, let's roll up our sleeves, or rather, get comfortable in our recliners, and start our path to better strength and flexibility.

THE SIGNIFICANCE OF STRENGTH AND FLEXIBILITY

Before we get into the exact postures and practices, let's first discuss why strength and flexibility are so essential, especially as we become older. Strength is required to preserve muscle mass, bone density, and general functional ability, hence preventing falls, accidents, and age-related reductions in physical function. Flexibility, on the other hand, is essential for preserving joint health, mobility, and range of motion while decreasing stiffness, tension, and the risk of injury. Together, strength and flexibility constitute the cornerstone of a healthy, active, and self-sufficient existence.

CHAIR YOGA POSES: STRENGTH AND FLEXIBILITY

Now, let's look at some chair yoga postures and sequences that are meant to help men over 50 gain strength and flexibility. These postures are gentle yet effective, providing a safe and accessible approach to test your body, build muscle endurance, and enhance joint mobility.

Remember to move thoughtfully and with awareness, respecting your body's limitations and making adjustments as needed to meet your own requirements and abilities.

CHAIR CAT-COW STRETCH.

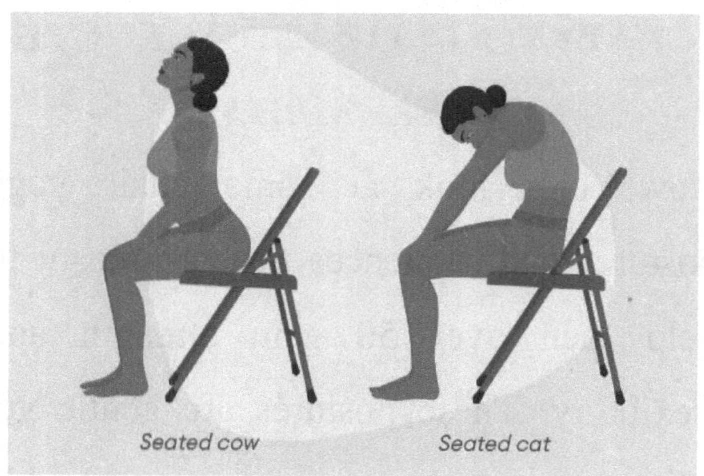

Begin by sitting tall in your chair, feet flat on the floor, hands resting on your knees. As you inhale, arch your back and elevate your chest to the ceiling, bringing your shoulder blades together and staring up. This is the cow pose. As you exhale, circle your back and bury your chin toward your chest, pulling your belly button towards your spine. This is a cat pose. Flow fluidly between Cow and Cat, connecting your movements with your breathing and allowing the stretch to pass into your spine and back muscles.

SEATED FORWARD FOLD WITH CHEST EXPANSION.

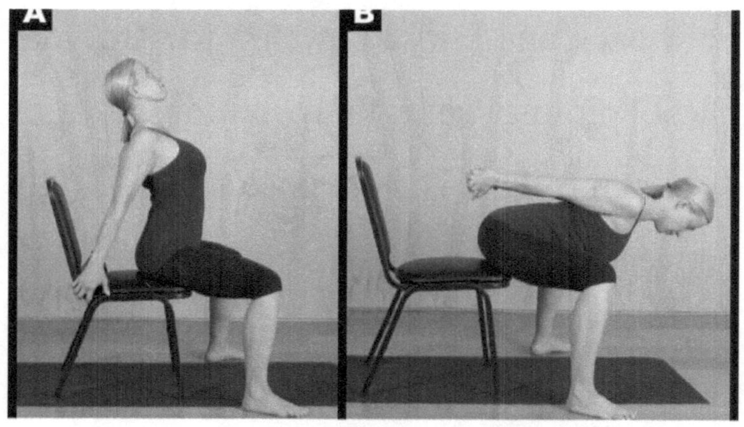

Begin by sitting tall in your chair, feet flat on the floor, hands resting on your thighs. As you inhale, extend through the crown of your head, and as you exhale, hinge forward from the hips, bringing your chest to your thighs and stretching your hands to your feet. Maintain a long spine and a calm neck as you fold forward, experiencing the stretch in your hamstrings and lower back. To deepen the stretch, interlace your fingers behind your back and slowly raise your arms upward to expand your chest and shoulders.

SEATED TWIST.

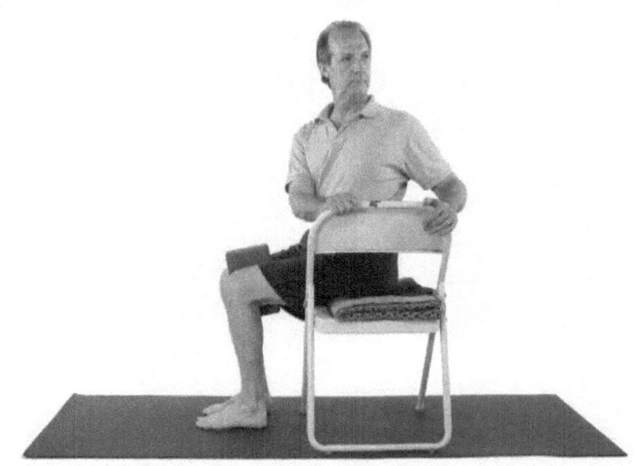

Sit tall in your chair, feet level on the floor, hands resting on your thighs. Inhale deeply, stretching your spine, then exhale and rotate to the right, resting your left hand on the outside of your right knee and your right hand on the back of the chair. Keep your spine long and your Your shoulders will relax as you slowly deepen the twist with each breath, experiencing the stretch in your spine, shoulders, and chest. Hold the twist for a few breaths before repeating on the opposite side.

CHAIR WARRIOR I

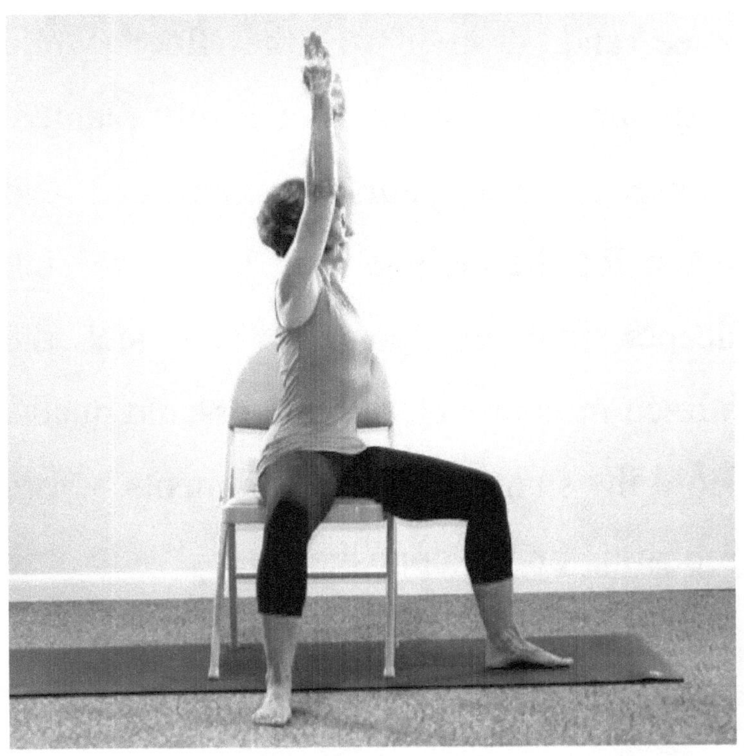

Begin by sitting tall in your chair, feet flat on the floor, hands resting on your thighs. As you inhale, raise your right leg off the ground and stretch it straight out in front of you, flexing your foot and working your quadriceps. As you exhale, bend your right knee and drop it to the floor while maintaining your left foot firmly planted. Inhale to raise your arms upwards and reach for the ceiling, then exhale to sink deeper into the position and feel the stretch in your right hip flexors and quads. Hold the stance for a few moments before repeating on the opposite side.

CHAIR WARRIOR 2

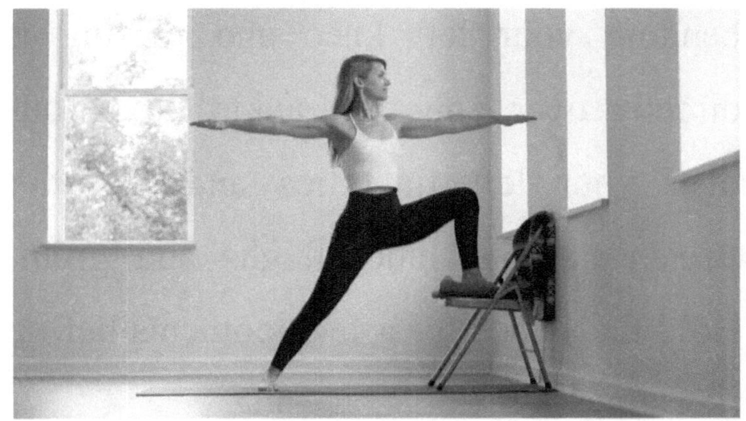

Sit tall in your chair, feet level on the floor, hands resting on your thighs. Inhale deeply, then exhale by stepping your right foot back behind you and rotating it 90 degrees to the side. Keep your left foot firmly planted on the ground and your hips square to the front of the chair. Inhale to elevate your arms parallel to the floor, extending out to the sides, and exhale to lower yourself into a lunge stance, bending your left knee and placing it directly over your left ankle. Look out over your left fingertips and feel the stretch in your inner thighs and groin. Hold the stance for a few moments before repeating on the opposite side.

CHAIR MOUNTAIN POSE

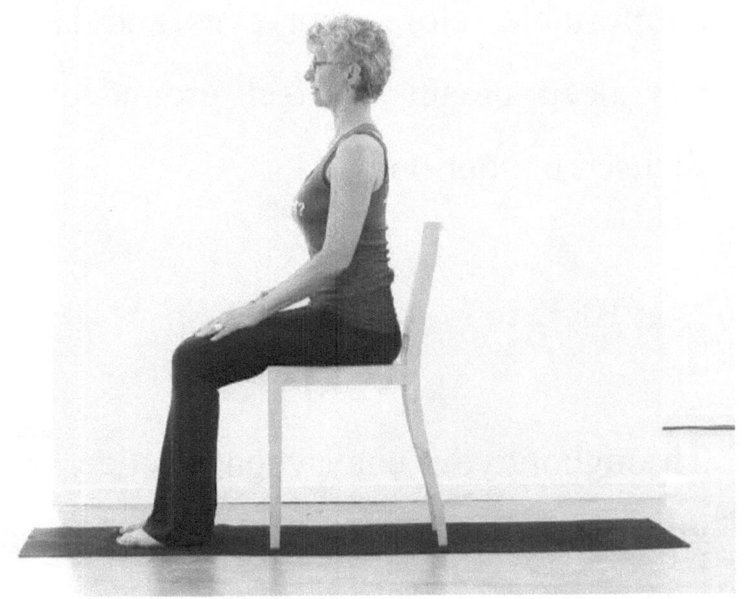

Begin by sitting tall in your chair, feet flat on the floor, hands resting on your thighs. Inhale deeply, stretching your spine, and then exhale, rooting down through your feet and seeing yourself growing tall and powerful like a mountain. Lift your chest using your core muscles, rotating your shoulders back and down. If you feel comfortable, close your eyes and take a few deep breaths to feel grounded and focused in your body.

BREATH AWARENESS AND MOVEMENT

Throughout your chair yoga practice, keep your breath in tune with your movement. Inhale deeply as you extend or lengthen, then exhale completely as you contract or release. By combining breath and movement, you may improve the flow of energy throughout your body, deepen your stretch, and build a sense of peace and focus in your mind. Maintain a smooth, steady, and regular breathing pattern as you go through each position and transition.

MINDFUL AWARENESS

Maintain conscious awareness during your chair yoga practice, paying attention to the sensations in your body, the rhythm of your breath, and the quality of your thoughts and emotions. Identify any areas of tension or pain and gradually explore techniques to release and soften, achieving ease and relaxation in each position. Develop a sense of curiosity and openness, enabling oneself to be completely present in the moment, free of judgment or expectation.

Chapter 3 has given us with a thorough examination of how chair yoga may assist men over 50 gain strength and flexibility. We've gone through a series of gentle postures and mindful movements to improve mobility, range of motion, and build a feeling of balance and stability in both the body and mind. Armed with these skills and strategies, we're ready to continue our path to better health, energy, and well-being via the transforming practice of chair yoga.

This chapter will provide you with the knowledge and practices you need to gain strength and flexibility via chair yoga.

CHAPTER 4

PAIN MANAGEMENT AND INJURY PREVENTION

In this chapter, we'll look at how chair yoga may help you manage pain, minimize discomfort, and avoid injury, particularly as you age. We'll use a variety of gentle postures, mindful movements, and relaxation methods to relieve common aches and pains, increase mobility, and promote overall well-being. So, let us roll up our sleeves, or rather, sit comfortably in our recliners, and begin our path to better comfort and vitality.

UNDERSTANDING PAIN AND DISCOMFORT.

Before we get into specific pain management and injury prevention measures, let's first define pain and discomfort, particularly as they pertain to aging. Our bodies change as we age, with muscles weakening, joints stiffening, and the chance of injury or chronic illnesses increasing. This might cause discomfort, stiffness, or soreness, affecting our ability to move, do everyday tasks, or engage in physical activity. Learning to listen to our body and respond with compassion and care allows us to begin to address these issues and find relief from pain and suffering.

GENTLE MOVEMENTS AND STRETCHING

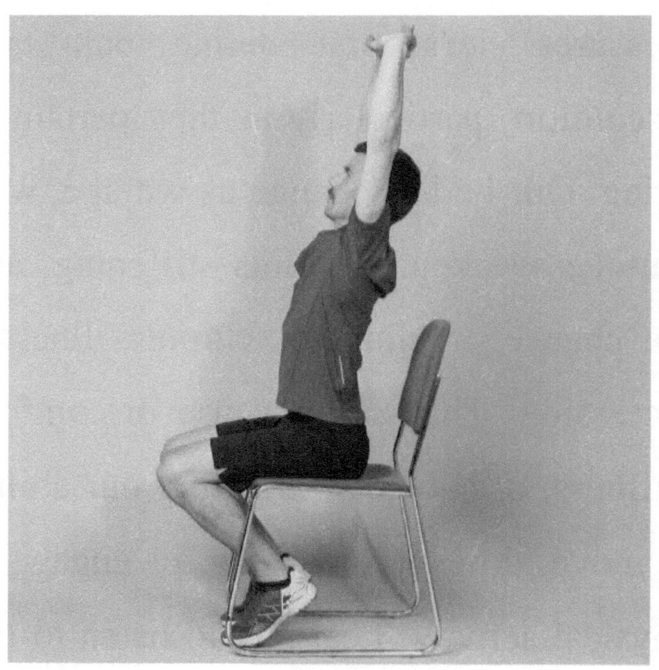

Gentle exercise and stretching are among the most effective techniques to manage discomfort and avoid damage. Chair yoga is a safe and easy approach to gently stretch and strengthen muscles, enhance joint mobility, and expand range of motion—all without putting excessive stress or pressure on the body. We can assist relieve tension, reduce stiffness, and increase general comfort and well-being by engaging in a series of moderate postures and exercises.

SEATED NECK STRETCHES

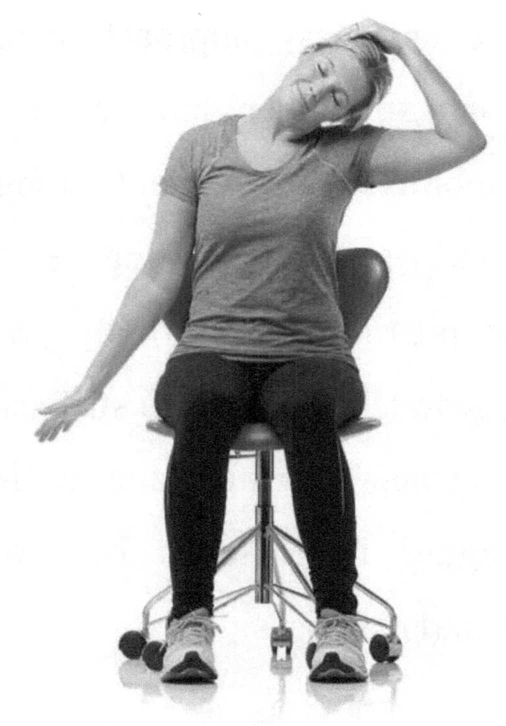

Begin by sitting tall in your chair, feet flat on the floor, hands resting on your thighs. Inhale and stretch through the top of your head. Exhale and gradually tilt your head to the right, bringing your right ear closer to your right shoulder. Hold this stretch for a few breaths, noticing the extending sensation on the left side of your neck. Repeat on the opposite side, turning your head to the left and placing your left ear near your left shoulder. Continue to change sides, moving gently and deliberately with your breathing.

SEATED SHOULDER ROLLS

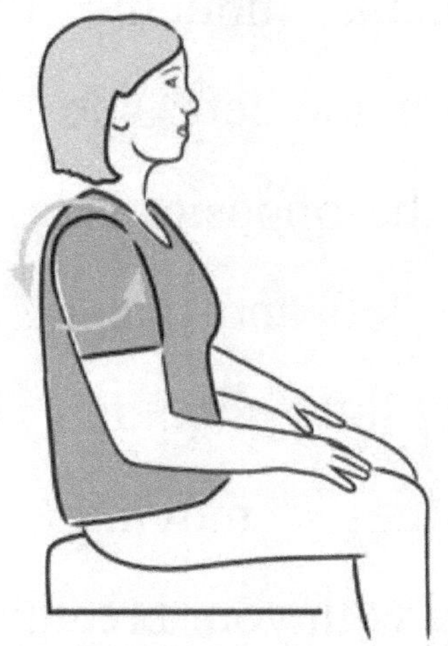

Sit tall in your chair, feet level on the
floor, hands resting on your thighs. Inhale
deeply, then exhale by rolling your
shoulders up and down in a smooth,
circular motion. Repeat this movement a
few times, letting your breath dictate the
rhythm. Take note of any areas of tension
or stiffness in your shoulders, and work on

releasing and relaxing them with each roll. Take your time and move mindfully, respecting your body's requirements and limitations.

SEATED SPINAL TWISTS.

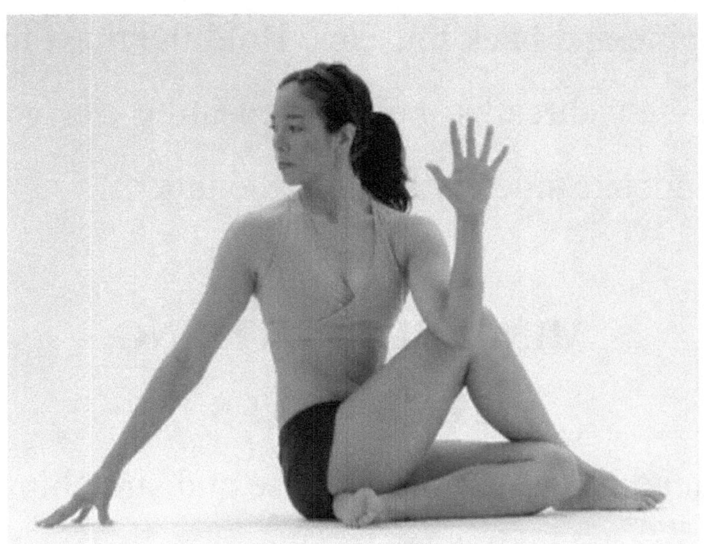

Begin by sitting tall in your chair, feet flat on the floor, hands resting on your thighs. Inhale deeply, then rotate to the right while exhaling, resting your left hand on the outside of your right knee and your right hand on the chair's back. Keep your spine extended and your shoulders relaxed as you gradually deepen the twist with each breath, feeling the stretch in your spine and back muscles. Hold the twist for a few breaths before repeating on the opposite side, twisting to the left.

MINDFUL BREATHING TECHNIQUES

In addition to mild exercise and stretching, mindfulness-based breathing practices can aid in the management of pain and discomfort. Focusing on the breath and establishing a sense of presence and awareness in the body can help to reduce stress, promote relaxation, and relieve muscular and joint stiffness. Deep belly breathing, ujjayi breath, or alternative nostril breathing can help to relax the nervous system, quiet the mind, and comfort the body.

PROGRESSIVE MUSCLE RELAXATION

Progressive muscle relaxation is another powerful pain relief and relaxation strategy. This is methodically tensing and releasing various muscle groups throughout the body, which helps to relieve stress, reduce muscular stiffness, and improve general relaxation. Begin by sitting comfortably in your chair and taking a few deep breaths to ground yourself. Then, starting with your feet, gradually work your way up your body, tensing each muscle group for a few seconds before releasing and relaxing entirely.

VISUALIZATION MEDITATION

Finally, let's look at visualization meditation as a strong pain and discomfort management technique. Take a few long breaths to calm and focus yourself. If you're feeling relaxed, close your eyes and envision yourself in a beautiful, serene setting—a placid beach, a verdant forest, or a quiet mountainside. Allow yourself to experience a sensation of serenity and relaxation pour over you, wrapping you in a warm hug of comfort and well-being.

Chapter 4 has taught us a range of pain-management and injury-prevention tactics using chair yoga. Gentle movement, stretching, mindfulness methods, and relaxation exercises can all assist to relieve discomfort, decrease stress, and increase general well-being. Armed with these skills and approaches, we can take control of our health and enjoy life to the fullest, regardless of age or physical ability.

CHAPTER 5

CHAIR YOGA FOR STRESS RELIEF AND MENTAL WELL-BEING.

In this chapter, we'll look at how chair yoga may help reduce stress, promote relaxation, and improve mental health. We'll use a variety of gentle postures, mindful movements, and relaxation methods to calm the mind, reduce anxiety, and build a sense of peace and serenity in both body and mind. So, let's get comfortable in our recliners and begin our path to better stress alleviation and mental health.

UNDERSTANDING STRESS AND ITS EFFECTS

Before we get into particular chair yoga techniques for stress reduction, let's first discuss the nature of stress and how it affects our entire health and well-being. Stress is the body's natural response to difficult or hazardous conditions, resulting in a cascade of physiological and psychological reactions. While acute stress can be useful in helping us respond to urgent dangers and challenges, chronic or extended stress can be harmful to our physical, emotional, and mental health, causing symptoms such as anxiety, despair, and exhaustion.

THE ADVANTAGES OF CHAIR YOGA FOR STRESS RELIEF

Chair yoga takes a comprehensive approach to stress management, treating the physical, mental, and emotional elements of stress with gentle movement, breath awareness, and relaxation methods. By practicing chair yoga on a daily basis, we may help quiet the nervous system, lower stress hormone production, and promote relaxation and well-being in both the body and mind. Chair yoga is accessible to people of all ages and fitness levels, making it an excellent practice for anybody wishing to reduce stress and improve their overall well-being.

GENTLE MOVEMENT AND BREATHING AWARENESS

Gentle movement mixed with breath awareness is an important aspect of chair yoga for stress alleviation. Synchronizing our movement with our breath can help to quiet the mind, improve our connection to the present moment, and produce a sensation of relaxation and comfort in the body. As we progress through each position, we'll concentrate on smooth, flowing motions led by the rhythm of our breath, letting tension and stress dissolve away with each exhale.

SEATED CAT-COW STRETCH

Begin by sitting tall in your chair, feet flat on the floor, hands resting on your thighs. As you inhale, arch your back and elevate your chest to the ceiling, bringing your shoulder blades together and staring up. This is the cow pose. As you exhale, circle your back and bury your chin toward your chest, pulling your belly button towards your spine. This is a cat pose. Flow fluidly between Cow and Cat, connecting your movements with your breathing and allowing the stretch to pass into your spine and back muscles.

SEATED FORWARD FOLD AND SHOULDER STRETCH

Begin by sitting tall in your chair, feet flat on the floor, hands resting on your thighs. As you inhale, extend through the crown of your head, and as you exhale, hinge forward from the hips, bringing your chest to your thighs and stretching your hands to your feet. Maintain a long spine and a calm neck as you fold forward, experiencing the stretch in your hamstrings and lower back. To deepen the stretch, interlace your fingers behind your back and slowly raise your arms upward to expand your chest and shoulders.

SEATED TWIST AND SIDE STRETCH

Sit tall in your chair, feet level on the floor, hands resting on your thighs. Inhale deeply, stretching your spine, then exhale and rotate to the right, resting your left hand on the outside of your right knee and your right hand on the back of the chair. Keep your spine extended and your shoulders relaxed as you gradually deepen the twist with each breath, feeling the stretch in your spine and back muscles. Hold the twist for a few breaths, then inhale to stretch your spine before exhaling to release and swap sides.

MINDFUL BREATHING TECHNIQUES

In addition to mild exercise, focused breathing practices can aid promote relaxation and stress reduction. Focusing on the breath and building a sense of presence and awareness in the body can help to quiet the mind, relax the nervous system, and foster a sense of peace and tranquility. Deep belly breathing, ujjayi breath, or alternate nostril breathing can help to settle the mind, deepen relaxation, and produce a sense of inner peace and well-being.

PROGRESSIVE MUSCLE RELAXATION

Progressive muscular relaxation is another powerful stress-relieving approach. This is methodically tensing and releasing various muscle groups throughout the body, which helps to relieve stress, reduce muscular stiffness, and improve general relaxation. Begin by sitting comfortably in your chair and taking a few deep breaths to ground yourself. Then, starting with your feet, gradually work your way up your body, tensing each muscle group for a few seconds before releasing and relaxing entirely.

VISUALIZATION MEDITATION

Finally, let's look at visualization meditation as a strong technique for stress alleviation and relaxation. Take a few long breaths to calm and focus yourself. If you're feeling relaxed, close your eyes and envision yourself in a beautiful, serene setting—a placid beach, a verdant forest, or a quiet mountainside. Allow yourself to experience a sensation of serenity and relaxation pour over you, wrapping you in a warm hug of comfort and well-being.

Chapter 5 has introduced us to a number of chair yoga practices and approaches for stress alleviation and mental health. Incorporating moderate movement, breath awareness, and relaxation techniques into our everyday routines can help calm the mind, reduce anxiety, and improve general relaxation and well-being. Armed with these skills and practices, we may take control of our mental health and live a more relaxed, resilient, and peaceful existence.

.

CHAPTER 6:

CHAIR YOGA TO ADDRESS SPECIFIC HEALTH CONCERNS

Welcome to the sixth chapter of "Flexibility at Any Age: Chair Yoga for Men Over 50." In this chapter, we'll look at how chair yoga may be adjusted to treat particular health issues and ailments that are frequent among men over 50. From arthritis and back pain to diabetes and heart disease, chair yoga is a safe and effective approach to manage symptoms, enhance function, and promote overall health. So let's look at how chair yoga might help you address your individual health challenges and achieve peak health and vitality.

ARTHRITIS RELIEF.

Arthritis is a common ailment marked by joint inflammation and stiffness, which can cause discomfort and limit movement. Chair yoga provides mild movement and stretching techniques that can help arthritis patients reduce pain and improve joint function. Regular chair yoga practice can assist to develop flexibility, reduce stiffness, and increase range of motion in afflicted joints, therefore alleviating pain and improving overall quality of life.

SEATED KNEE TO CHEST STRETCH

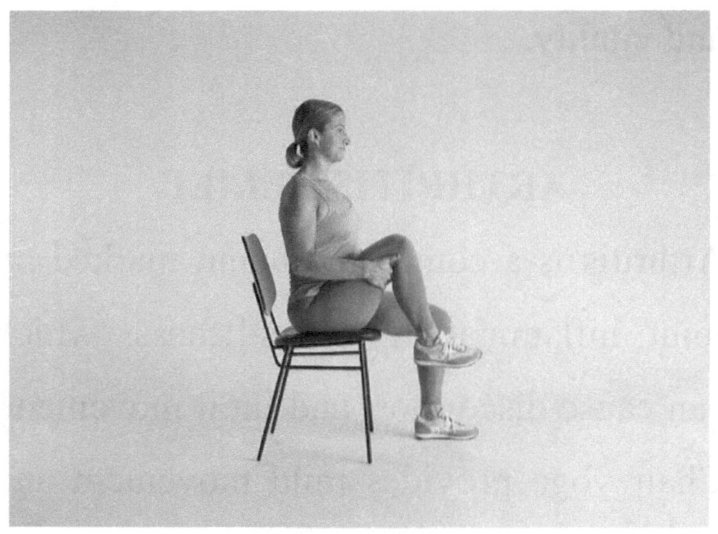

Begin by sitting tall in your chair, feet flat on the floor, hands resting on your thighs. Inhale deeply, and as you exhale, raise your right knee to your chest, wrapping your arms around your shin and gently dragging it into you. Hold the stretch for a few breaths, experiencing the relief in your hips and lower back, before releasing and switching sides. Repeat on the left side, raising your left knee to your chest and holding for a few breaths before letting go.

SEATED SHOULDER OPENER

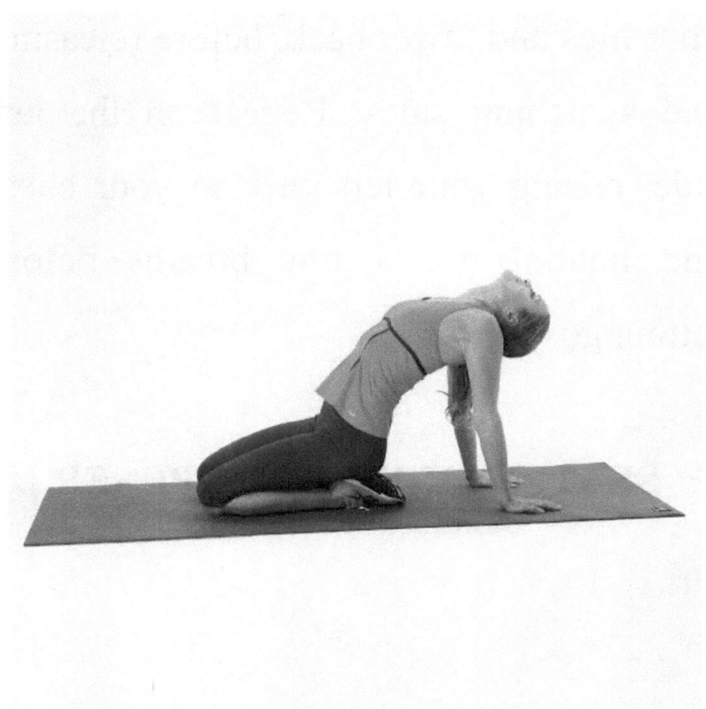

Sit tall in your chair, feet level on the floor, hands resting on your thighs. Inhale deeply and, as you exhale, extend your right arm across your body, resting your left hand on your elbow. Gently push your right arm on your left shoulder to feel the stretch in your shoulder and upper back. Hold the stretch for a few moments before releasing and switching sides, stretching your left arm across your body and pressing into your right shoulder.

DIABETES MANAGEMENT.

Diabetes is a chronic disorder characterized by elevated blood sugar levels, which can cause symptoms such as tiredness, thirst, and frequent urination. Chair yoga can help manage diabetes by encouraging relaxation, lowering stress, and boosting circulation and blood flow throughout the body. Incorporating mild exercise, breath awareness, and relaxation techniques into your daily routine can help manage blood sugar levels, increase insulin sensitivity, and boost overall well-being.

SEATED SIDE BEND.

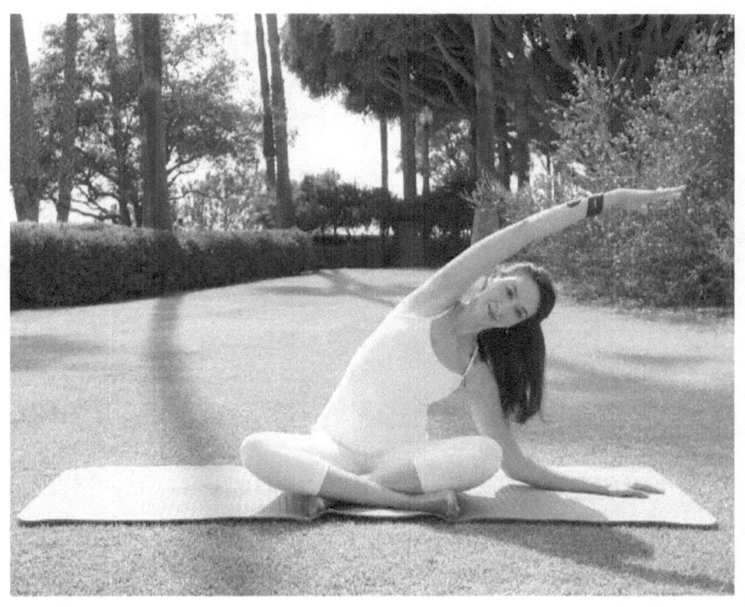

Begin by sitting tall in your chair, feet flat on the floor, hands resting on your thighs. Inhale deeply, and as you exhale, extend your right arm up to the sky, lengthening your fingertips. As you inhale, extend your spine, and as you exhale, lean gently to the left, feeling the stretch down your right side. Hold the stretch for a few breaths before inhaling to return to the center and repeating on the opposite side.

HEART HEALTH SUPPORT

Heart disease is the biggest cause of mortality in males over the age of 50, and risk factors include high blood pressure, high cholesterol, and a sedentary lifestyle. Chair yoga can be extremely beneficial to heart health by increasing relaxation, lowering stress, and enhancing cardiovascular function. Regular chair yoga practice can help lower blood pressure, cut cholesterol levels, and strengthen the heart muscle, all of which minimize the risk of heart disease and improve cardiovascular health.

SEATED HEART OPENING POSE

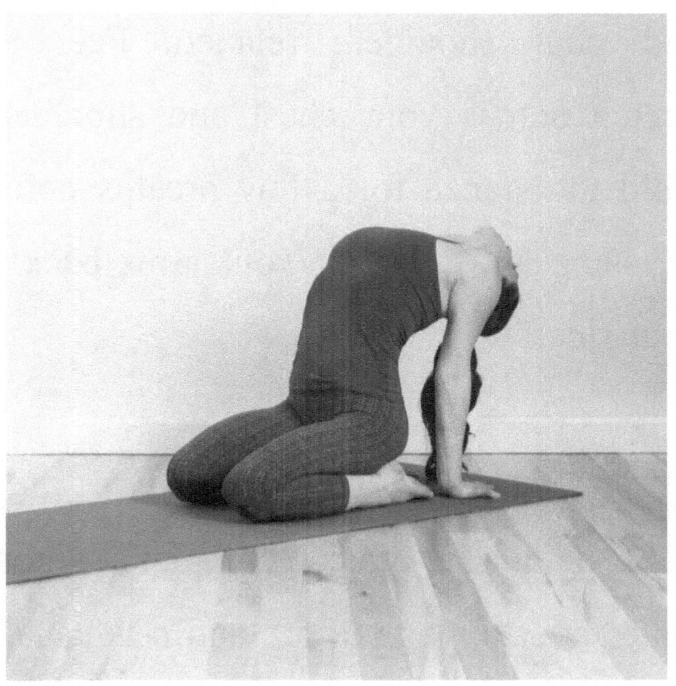

Sit tall in your chair, feet level on the floor, hands resting on your thighs. Inhale deeply, then as you exhale, interlace your fingers behind your back, pulling your shoulder blades together and opening your chest to the ceiling. As you gradually elevate your chest, keep your spine long and your shoulders relaxed. Feel the stretch across your chest and shoulders. Hold the stance for a few breaths before releasing and relaxing your arms back to your sides.

BACK PAIN RELIEF

Back pain is a typical complaint among males over the age of 50, and it is usually caused by bad posture, muscular imbalances, or degenerative changes in the spine. Chair yoga combines mild stretching and strengthening movements to help relieve back pain and enhance spinal health. Regular chair yoga practice can help you gain flexibility, reduce muscular tension, and improve posture, resulting in less discomfort and better function in your back and spine.

SEATED SPINAL TWIST.

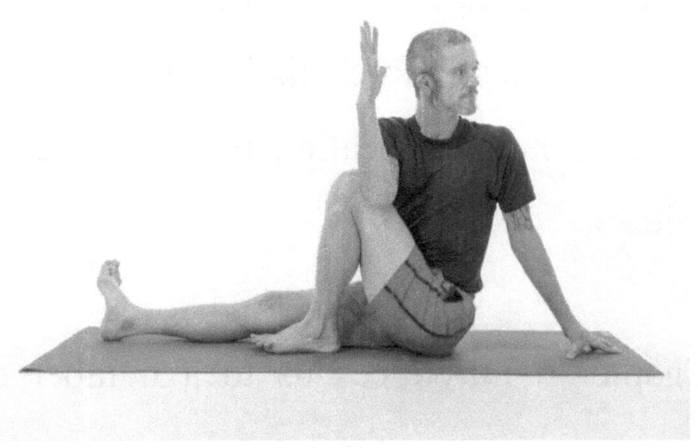

Begin by sitting tall in your chair, feet flat on the floor, hands resting on your thighs. Inhale deeply, then rotate to the right while exhaling, resting your left hand on the outside of your right knee and your right hand on the chair's back. Keep your spine extended and your shoulders relaxed as you gradually deepen the twist with each breath, feeling the stretch in your spine and back muscles. Hold the twist for a few breaths before inhaling to return to the center and repeating on the opposite side.

Chapter 6 introduces us to a number of chair yoga practices and approaches designed to address particular health conditions common among men over the age of 50. Whether you have arthritis, diabetes, heart disease, or back pain, chair yoga provides a safe and effective technique to manage symptoms, enhance function, and promote overall wellness. Armed with these skills and approaches, you can take control of your health and live your life to the fullest, regardless of any health issues you may face.

CHAPTER 7:

INCORPORATING CHAIR YOGA INTO DAILY LIFE

Welcome to chapter 7 of "Flexibility at Any Age: Chair Yoga for Men Over 50." In this chapter, we will look at practical ways to incorporate chair yoga into your daily life. We'll cover everything from setting up a dedicated practice room to adding chair yoga into your regular routine. So let's get started and see how you may benefit from chair yoga every day, no matter where you are.

CREATING A DEDICATED PRACTICE SPACE

One of the first stages in incorporating chair yoga into your daily routine is to set up a designated practice area where you can practice comfortably and securely. Choose a calm, clutter-free location in your house to set up your chair and any supports you might require, such as a yoga mat, blocks, or blankets. Make sure the space is well-lit and ventilated, with plenty of room to move about in all directions. Consider using some soothing materials, such as candles, plants, or quiet music, to improve your practice environment and generate a sense of serenity and relaxation.

SETTING A DAILY ROUTINE

To incorporate chair yoga into your everyday life, you must develop a consistent practice regimen that works for you. Set up a certain time each day to practice chair yoga, whether it's first thing in the morning, during your lunch break, or before bed. By including chair yoga into your everyday routine, you'll find it easier to stay engaged and motivated, and you'll see the results of your practice sooner. Remember, even a few minutes of chair yoga every day may significantly improve your general health and well-being.

STARTING SMALL AND GAINING MOMENTUM

If you're new to chair yoga or have a hectic schedule, it's fine to start slowly and develop momentum over time. Begin with short, reasonable practice sessions of 10-15 minutes each day, gradually increasing the time and intensity as you gain comfort and confidence. Remember, consistency is essential, so make your practice a regular habit, even if it's only for a few minutes each day. Starting small and gradually developing momentum increases your chances of sticking with your practice and reaping long-term advantages.

IMPLEMENTING CHAIR YOGA THROUGHOUT THE DAY

One of the most appealing aspects of chair yoga is that it can be done at any time and from any location, making it simple to include into your daily routine. Look for ways to include chair yoga into your daily routine, whether it's at your desk, in the kitchen, or while watching TV. While seated in your chair, you can perform easy stretches, breathing exercises, or mindfulness practices to help decrease stress, enhance energy, and improve concentration and productivity. Get creative and discover methods to include chair yoga into your regular activities, making it a natural part of your routine.

PRACTICE MINDFUL MOVEMENT AND BREATH AWARENESS

As you go about your day, use mindful movement and breath awareness to be grounded, present, and focused. Pay attention to your posture, alignment, and breathing whether walking, standing, or sitting, and make tiny modifications as needed to encourage comfort and ease in your body. Identify any areas of tension or pain and carefully explore techniques to release and soften, resulting in increased relaxation and ease with each breath. By incorporating mindful movement and breath awareness into your daily routine, you may create a feeling of mindfulness and presence in your life, reducing stress, increasing awareness, and improving overall well-being.

CONNECTING WITH THE COMMUNITY AND SUPPORT

Finally, try joining a community or support group for those who are interested in chair yoga and holistic health. Connecting with others, whether through a local yoga class, participation in online forums or social media groups, or attendance at seminars and retreats, may give vital support, encouragement, and inspiration on your path. Share your experiences, ask questions, and provide support to others as you navigate your chair yoga practice and discover new ways to incorporate it into your everyday life. Building a supportive community can help you stay committed to your practice and connect with yourself and others.

Chapter 7 has given us practical ideas for incorporating chair yoga into our daily lives. We can make chair yoga a sustainable and enjoyable part of our lifestyle by setting up a dedicated practice space, developing a daily routine, starting small and building momentum, incorporating chair yoga throughout the day, practicing mindful movement and breath awareness, and connecting with community and support. Armed with these tools and approaches, we may enjoy the advantages of chair yoga every day, no matter where we are.

CHAPTER 8

ADVANCED CHAIR YOGA PRACTICES

Welcome to chapter 8 of "Flexibility at Any Age: Chair Yoga for Men Over 50." In this chapter, we'll look at advanced chair yoga techniques that will challenge and deepen your practice while also providing new chances for development and discovery. From advanced postures,

From sequences to specific methods and modifications, these practices will help you broaden your horizons and elevate your chair yoga practice to new heights.

So, let us dive in and explore the potential of advanced chair yoga.

DISCOVERING ADVANCED POSES AND SEQUENCES

Advanced chair yoga postures and sequences provide additional challenges and chances for growth while strengthening the body, increasing flexibility, and deepening awareness and focus. Advanced poses, which range from balancing poses and inversions to deep stretches and backbends, need more strength, stability, and attention, as well as a desire to experiment and push yourself beyond your comfort zone. Incorporating difficult poses and sequences into your practice can help you develop resilience, courage, and confidence both on and off the mat.

CHAIR WARRIOR III

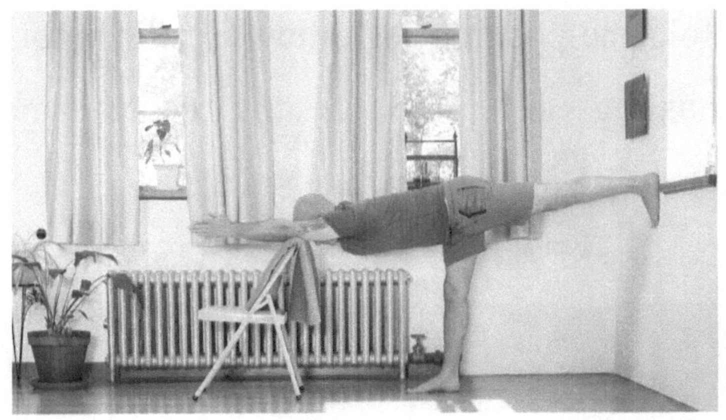

Begin by sitting tall in your chair, feet flat on the floor, hands resting on your thighs. Inhale deeply, and as you exhale, shift your weight to your left foot, raising your right foot off the floor and stretching straight back behind you. Keep your spine long and your core engaged as you tilt forward from your hips, bringing your torso parallel to the ground and stretching your arms forward in line with your ears. Hold the position for a few breaths before inhaling to return to the center and repeating on the opposite side.

SEATED PIGEON POSE

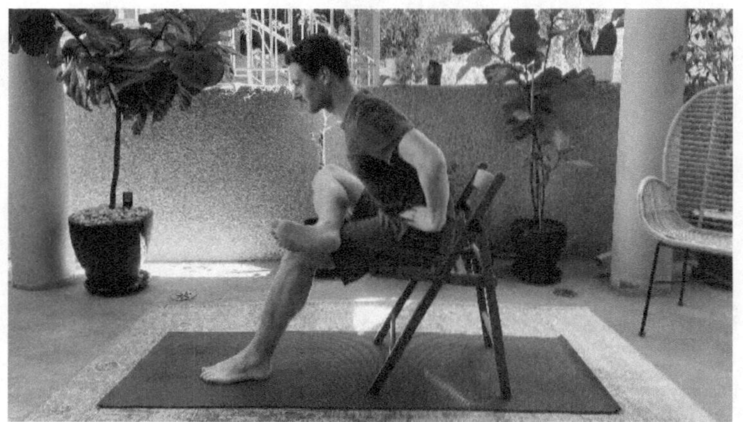

Begin by sitting tall in your chair, feet flat on the floor, hands resting on your thighs.

Inhale deeply, then exhale, crossing your right ankle over your left knee and flexing your right foot to protect the knee. Maintain a long spine and an elevated chest while gently pressing down on your right knee with your right hand, feeling the stretch in your right hip and glute. Hold for a few breaths before releasing and switching sides, crossing your left ankle over your right knee and repeating the stretch on the opposite side.

CHAIR HALF MOON POSE

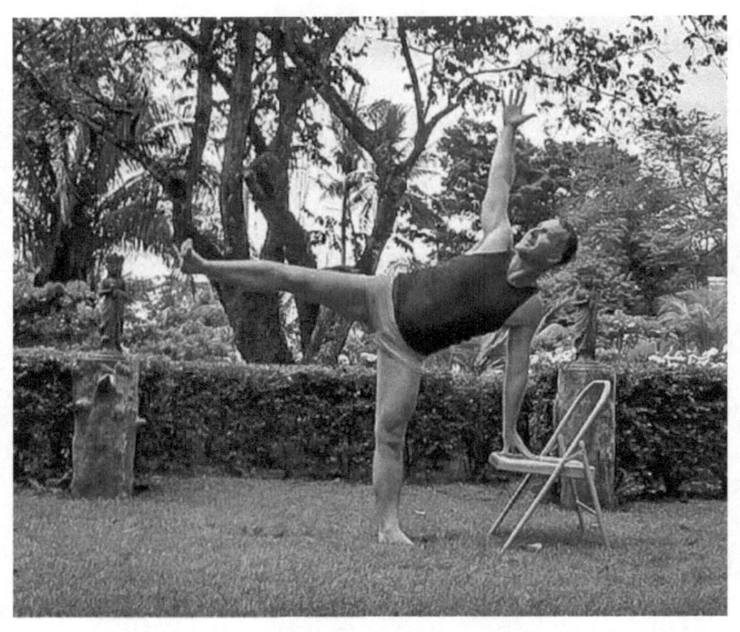

Begin by sitting tall in your chair, feet flat on the floor, hands resting on your thighs. Inhale deeply, then exhale by extending your right leg out to the side, keeping your foot flexed and your toes facing forward. Press down with your left foot and extend your right arm forward and over to the left, forming a long line of energy from your left foot to your right fingertips. Hold the position for a few breaths before inhaling to return to the center and repeating on the opposite side.

SPECIALIZED TECHNIQUES AND VARIATIONS

In addition to advanced poses and sequences, specific methods and modifications can help improve your chair yoga practice by providing fresh perspectives and approaches to established poses and motions. These approaches, which range from pranayama (breathwork) and meditation to restorative yoga and yoga nidra, can assist to deepen relaxation, promote healing, and create a sense of inner calm and wellbeing. By experimenting with particular approaches and variations, you will uncover new aspects to your practice and unleash hidden potential in yourself.

SEATED BREATH OF FIRE

Sit tall in your chair, feet level on the floor, hands resting on your thighs. Inhale deeply through your nose, filling your lungs with air; then, expel strongly through your nose, pushing your belly in and out with each breath. Continue to breathe quickly and regularly, concentrating on the movement of your abdomen and the sensation of air moving into and out of your nostrils. Practice for 1-3 minutes, then release and resume regular breathing.

SEATED GUIDED VISUALIZATION

Close your eyes and take a few deep breaths to calm and focus yourself. As you breathe in, visualize a brilliant, warm light filling your body with energy and vigor, beginning at the top of your head and going down to your toes. As you exhale, visualize all of your tension and stress melting away, leaving you peaceful, relaxed, and at peace. Continue to envision this healing light streaming through your body, nourishing and renewing every cell and fiber of your being, until you are fully calm and comfortable.

CHAIR YOGA ADVANCED BALANCE AND STABILITY

Advanced balance and stability poses test your coordination, focus, and proprioception, which helps to enhance balance and prevent falls. By performing advanced balance poses on a daily basis, you will develop the muscles of the core, legs, and feet while also improving your attention and awareness. Advanced balance postures, which range from standing on one leg to balancing on your hands or forearms, provide limitless opportunities for physical and mental development.

SEATED TREE POSE

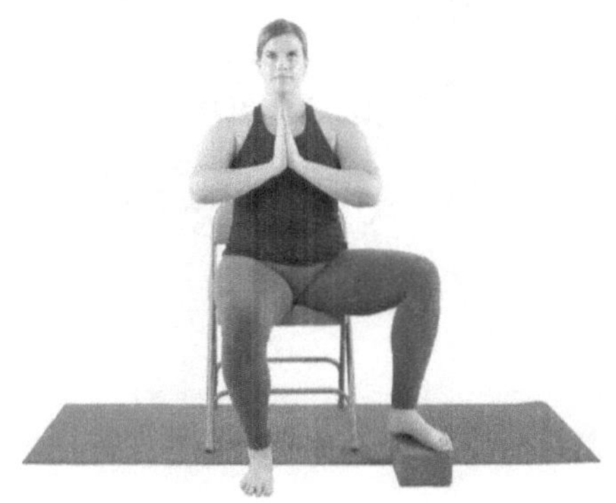

Begin by sitting tall in your chair, feet flat on the floor, hands resting on your thighs. Inhale deeply, then exhale while lifting your right foot off the floor and placing the sole on the inner of your left leg, just above the knee. Press your foot into your thigh, and your thigh into your foot, to achieve stability and balance in the position. Bring your hands to a prayer posture at your heart's center, or stretch your arms upwards for an additional challenge. Hold the position for a few breaths before releasing and switching sides

CONCLUSION

In this thorough guide to chair yoga for men over 50, we've looked at a variety of practices, methods, and ideas to help you improve your flexibility, strength, balance, and general health. Chair yoga provides a varied and accessible approach to fitness and mindfulness, with everything from mild stretches and breathing exercises to advanced postures and specialized methods that may be adapted to your own requirements and preferences.

Throughout this trip, we've learnt the value of mindfulness and present in our practice, focusing on our breath, body, and mind as we progress through each posture and sequence. Staying present and engaged in the moment allows us to develop our practice, improve our attention, and discover greater serenity and clarity inside ourselves.

We've also looked at the physical advantages of chair yoga, which include increased flexibility, strength and stability, better posture and alignment, and increased mobility and range of motion. Regular practice can help to develop the body's muscles, increase circulation and blood flow, and promote general physical health and well-being.

In addition to the physical advantages, chair yoga has several mental and emotional benefits, such as stress reduction, anxiety alleviation, improved mood and emotional control, and increased relaxation and sleep. By combining mindfulness methods, breathwork, and meditation into our practice, we may create a sense of inner calm, resilience, and well-being that lasts beyond the mat and into our daily lives.

As we get to the end of our trip, keep in mind that chair yoga is more than simply a physical practice; it is a comprehensive approach to health and wellbeing that includes the body, mind, and spirit. Whether you have physical restrictions, chronic health concerns, or simply want to enhance your overall quality of life, chair yoga is a safe, accessible, and effective approach to meet your health and fitness objectives.

So, as you continue your chair yoga adventure, remember to be patient and kind with yourself, acknowledging your body's limits while praising its strengths.

Accept the process of development and change, and believe that each step you take on the mat will bring you closer to greater health, energy, and well-being.

Thank you for joining me on this path, and may chair yoga continue to enhance your life in innumerable ways.